Women wit

Using your Exercise Ball

Lisa M. Wolfe

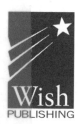

Wish Publishing
Terre Haute, Indiana
www.wishpublishing.com

Women with Balls © 2006 Lisa M. Wolfe

All rights reserved under International and Pan-American Copyright Conventions

No part of this book may be reproduced, stored in a data base or other retrieval system, or transmitted in any form, by any means, including mechanical, photocopy, recording or otherwise, without the prior written permission of the publisher.

LCCN: 2005936064

Editorial assistance provided by Dorothy Chambers and Cristina Gowrylow

Cover designed by Phil Velikan

Interior and cover photography by Morgan Wolfe at Ohana Karate

Printed in the United States of America
10 9 8 7 6 5 4 3 2 1

Published in the United States by
Wish Publishing
P.O. Box 10337
Terre Haute, IN 47801, USA
www.wishpublishing.com

For my mother, the strongest woman I know

Table of Contents

Preface

I hope it was the title that prompted you to pick this book. I admire that you have a desire to be a strong, confident woman with balls.

These exercises will guide you toward the physical strength you have been seeking. Along with the physical strength comes the mental confidence that you can do anything you dream of doing. One of my favorite mottos lately is, "If you can believe it, you can achieve it."

Your first step was opening this book. The next step is dedicating an hour a day to exercise. These ball exercises are fun and effective, so put away any excuses and start today. Believe that you can have the strength and confidence of which you have dreamed and you will achieve it.

I hope you find the workout you've been searching for and I wish you success in taking care of you!

In health,
Lisa

Introduction

Balls come in a variety of sizes, colors and textures. They have different uses, purposes and features. What do we do with them? How can this round shape provide an effective workout?

Stability Balls

Whether a stability ball was sitting in the corner of a gym, being used on an infomercial or waiting to be purchased on the store shelf, chances are you probably have seen one.

Stability balls are large, inflated, rubber balls that vary in size and color. The ball can be used as exercise equipment, a chair, or a training tool in physical education classes. As exercise equipment, the ball can be used in place of weights. This air-filled ball can also be used in place of a bench and provides an unstable, yet comfortable and supportive base for strength training exercises.

The greatest benefit to stability ball training is core strength. When exercising with a ball, the entire muscular system is activated in order to maintain posture and balance. As opposed to passive sitting on a chair or a bench, active sitting is required when sitting on a ball. The muscles of the spine work with the muscles of the stomach in order to stabilize the body. This

Ball Benefits
- improved posture
- spinal flexibility
- spinal stability
- disc decompression
- reduced risk for back injuries
- reduced back pain

Lisa M. Wolfe

> **Ball Benefits**
> - improved core strength
> - overall body strength
> - enhanced balance
> - increased flexibility
> - workout variety
> - ease of use

enhanced muscular coordination improves overall back health.

Proper use of the ball will improve your muscles' strength, tone and endurance. The large muscle groups and the smaller stabilizing muscles will gain strength. This is because multiple groups of muscles work together to create increased challenge in a ball workout. Specifically, this ball training workout will increase your weight loss, metabolism, muscular strength and muscular tone.

Flexibility is also enhanced through the addition of the ball into your stretching exercises. Using the ball allows your body to be manipulated deeper into stretching exercises by providing support for the joints. The ball is also a safer option for those who find discomfort when sitting on, and getting up from, the floor.

In all of the exercises, the ball requires the body to maintain perfect posture on an unstable surface. Whether sitting, kneeling, or laying on the ball, the body's balance is awakened.

Stability balls often have different names, such as fitness ball, exercise ball or Swiss ball. The manufacturers vary, from those who provide commercial grade balls to those who supply the at-home user. The main difference between the suppliers is the maximum weight the ball will support. Most balls will support between 700 and 1000 pounds.

When choosing a ball, look for one that is designed to hold your body's weight and is appropriate for your height. As a general guideline, for those under 5 feet tall, a 45 cm ball will provide the correct base. For those between 5 and 6 feet tall, a

55 cm ball will provide the correct base. If the balls do not have a measurement on them, the best way to gauge proper size is to sit on top of the ball. When you sit on the ball, the angles at the hips and the knees should both be 90 degrees. If your knees are bending too much, the ball is small. If your knees are straightening, the ball is large.

Medicine Balls

Medicine balls are intimidating for many people. The name alone is enough to cause trepidation. In the past, medicine balls have been associated with old black-and-white films of burly men throwing these sand-filled balls at each other.

This fear factor can be reduced when we realize that a medicine ball is simply a weighted ball filled with sand that is useful in upper and lower body training. They come in variable weight amounts to accommodate all levels of strength.

These balls can be used in place of dumbbells for many appropriate, fun and effective exercises. The ease of use, increased safety, and ability to maneuver through exercises that wouldn't be appropriate when using a dumbbell, add to the appeal of using a medicine ball. The act of grasping the medicine ball helps to improve hand, finger and wrist strength. The rubber ball is gentler than a metal dumbbell for those suffering from arthritis in the hands or carpal tunnel in the wrists.

> Ball Benefits
> - improved muscular strength
> - improved muscular tone
> - ease of use
> - increased variety of exercises

The balls can be purchased at any sporting goods store. The beginner should choose a 6- to 10-pound ball for proper resistance. The balls also vary from those with bounce to those

Lisa M. Wolfe

without bounce. The balls without the bounce will be best for the exercises included here.

Mini Xerballs

These mini, 4- to 6-inch Xerballs resemble small medicine balls. Being similar to medicine balls, they can also be used in place of dumbbells. The balls have a softer outer shell than a medicine ball, which makes them an easy partner with exercises such as yoga and Pilates. The balls fit comfortably in the hands which reduces stress to the fingers and wrists. Another benefit is that you can let go of the ball quickly during the workout if the resistance becomes too great, without risk of injury to your toes or other body parts. The balls are also extremely portable. You can place them in a bag, or take them with you to the gym or exercise class without the worry of dropping them.

Ball Benefits
- comfortable to use
- improved strength
- decreased risk of injury
- ease of partnering with other exercises
- portable
- durable

The balls are sold at sporting goods stores and super stores. The amount of weight should correspond with what you would use in a dumbbell weight. In general, a weight of 4 to 8 pounds will provide proper resistance.

The focus of the exercises in this book is muscular strength training. The more muscle tissue you have, the faster your metabolism will burn because your muscle tissue burns calories 24 hours a day. These exercises will help with weight loss yet become even more effective when combined with an aerobic exercise program. Examples of aerobic exercises are walking, jogging, cycling, swimming, ball bouncing, etc.

This workout can be used as a full-body strength training program to be performed every other day. You can also split the body up into segments to train one or two muscle groups at a time. A day of rest should follow that muscle's training day. For example: day one, strengthen the arms and chest; day two, strengthen the back, legs and shoulders.

Lisa M. Wolfe

The Warm-Up

Your body needs to be warm before participating in strength training exercises. The stability ball provides you a unique and fun way to warm up. The goal in the warm-up is to increase the heart rate and blood flow to the muscles. A warm muscle is less likely to suffer an injury than a cold muscle.

Prior to beginning, it is important to inflate the ball according to the manufacturer's instructions. It is safe to leave the ball slightly deflated, which will make the exercises easier. It is unsafe to overinflate the ball. This could cause the ball to explode. The ball should be firm for those who have prior use with and feel comfortable on the ball. Check your ball for proper fit and make sure you have clear space in which to move around. Due to the risk of falling, you want to be sure that furniture and other dangerous objects are pushed out of your way.

The ball should be used indoors and on carpet or smooth floor. You should wear workout clothing including shirts, pants and shoes. The shirt and pants help prevent sticking to the ball which could irritate the skin. Also, if the body becomes sweaty, a shirt prevents you from slipping off the ball.

Warm-Up Benefits

- prepares the muscles for the workout
- increases the heart rate
- improves blood circulation
- reduces risk of muscular injury
- allows time for the mind to focus on the workout

Lisa M. Wolfe

This warm-up consists of three to five minutes of various ball-bouncing actions. The movement is always on the bounce. For example, during knee lifting the feeling is: bounce with feet together, right knee lift, bounce, left knee lift, etc.

You can create your own movements based on your personal favorites. If you enjoy the twist, you can rotate your hips on the ball. If you like downhill skiing, you can mimic a mogul movement by shifting the feet and knees from side to side. There is no limit to the number of movements you can create, so let your imaginations run wild and have a great time exercising!

Bouncing

Begin by sitting on top of your stability ball. Your knees are bent at a 90-degree angle, with your feet on the floor in front of you. Keep your back straight by sitting up tall and pull your stomach in tight. Start gently bouncing up and down by pressing through your heels. The bounce is varied by increasing the intensity or the speed. The arms lift up and down overhead, out to the sides or in small bicep curls. Balance is helped by finding a focal point on a wall in front

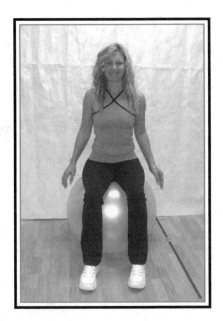

of you. Maintain normal breathing while you continue bouncing for two minutes.

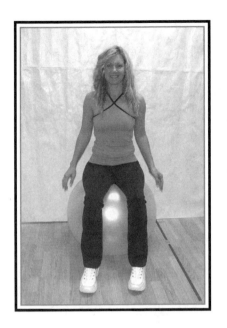 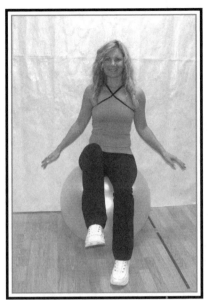

Knee Lifts

This is a continuation of the bounce. As the bouncing continues, we begin to alternate knee lifts on every other bounce. On the first bounce, both feet are on the floor. With the second bounce, the right foot lifts off the floor, bringing the knee toward the chest. On the third bounce, both feet are on the floor. With the fourth bounce, the left foot lifts off the floor, bringing the knee toward the chest. Continue alternating these knee lifts for one minute. For an advanced challenge, lift both knees at one time. The lift is still on every other bounce: the first bounce, both feet are on the floor; the next bounce, both feet are lifted. Repeat.

Lisa M. Wolfe

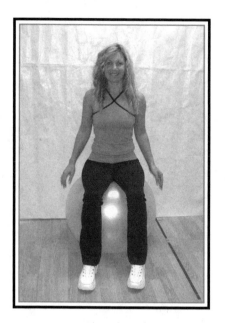 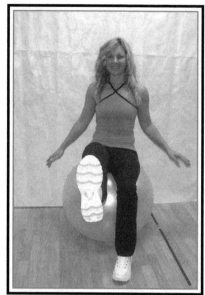

Kicks

The kicks progress from the knee lifts. Instead of lifting a bent leg, we now straighten the leg to the front for a kick. On the first bounce, both feet are on the floor. With the second bounce, the right foot lifts off the floor and the leg extends away from the body.On the third bounce, both feet are on the floor. With the fourth bounce, the left foot lifts off the floor extending the leg. Continue alternating these kicks for one minute. For an advanced challenge, kick both legs at the same time. This movement uses a strong core and solid balance.On the first bounce, both feet are on the floor. On the next bounce, both legs are extended. Repeat.

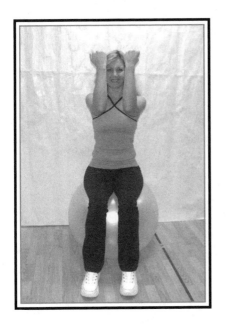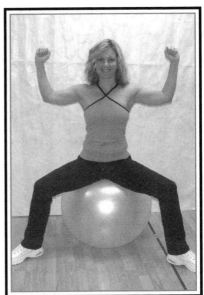

Jumping Jacks

Begin by bouncing with the knees and feet close together in front of the body. Bend the arms at the elbows and place the palms in front of the face. Bounce One is this closed position of a jumping jack. For Bounce Two, open the legs and arms out to the sides. Bounce Three, close. Bounce Four, open. Continue alternating this closed and open jack for one minute. For an advanced challenge, increase the speed or intensity of the bounce.

Lisa M. Wolfe

Stability Ball Strengthening Exercises

These stability ball exercises use the ball and the weight of your body to provide strength training benefits. Each exercise should be executed slowly and with muscular control. A faster movement relies on momentum and not muscular contraction.

Guidelines

- Repeat 10 to 12 repetitions of each exercise.
- Perform two to three sets for maximum strength gains.
- Keep the spine straight and the stomach muscles pulled in tight.
- Maintain a firm grasp on the ball. Refrain from gripping too tightly.
- Keep a slight bend in the knees for standing exercises.
- Keep a slight bend in the elbows throughout the exercises.

Lisa M. Wolfe

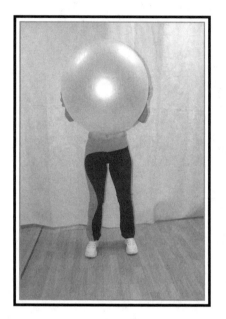 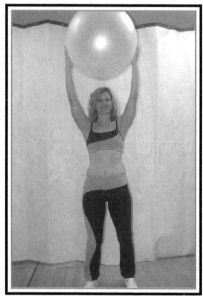

Overhead Press

Stand tall with feet hip-distance apart. Hold onto the ball with both hands and place ball onto chest with elbows bent. Exhale and lift the arms overhead. Keep a slight bend in the elbows. Inhale and release the ball back to the chest.

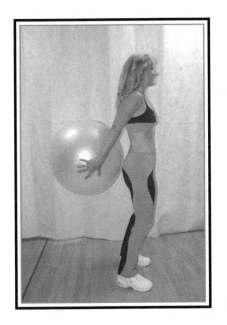 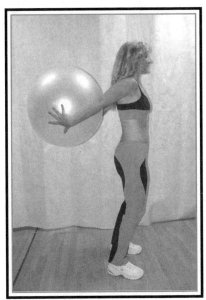

Rear Shoulder Lift

Stand tall with feet hip-distance apart. Hold onto the ball with both hands and place ball onto lower back. Exhale and lift the straight arms toward the ceiling. Keep the spine tall and refrain from leaning forward. Inhale and release the ball to the lower back.

Lisa M. Wolfe

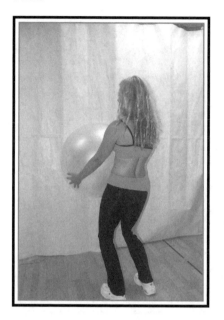 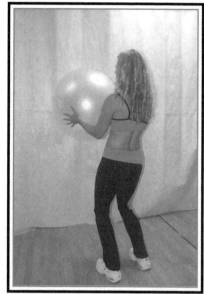

Wall Rolls

Stand facing a wall with feet hip-distance apart. Place the ball onto the wall at the level of your hips. Place hands underneath the ball. Exhale and bend the elbows, rolling the ball up the wall. Keep the elbows pressed into the rib cage. Press into the ball as you are rolling to increase the resistance. Inhale and straighten the arms, releasing the ball to the start position.

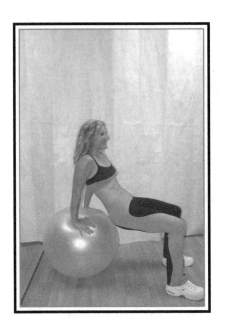
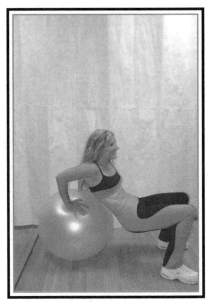

Dips

Sit on top of the ball. Place your hands on the ball next to your hips. Point your fingers toward your legs, as opposed to behind the body. Keep your arms straight and walk your feet away from the ball, moving your hips off the ball. Keep the knees bent. Inhale and bend your elbows, lowering hips toward the floor. Point the elbows straight behind the body. Exhale and straighten the elbows, raising the hips off the floor. For an intermediate movement, straighten the legs. For an advanced movement, place the heel of one foot onto the toes of the other.

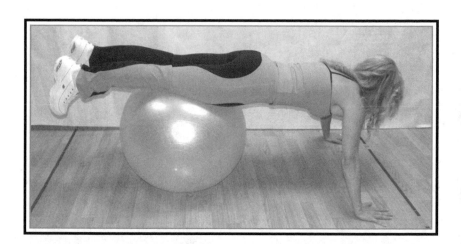

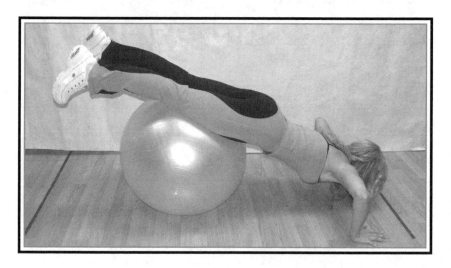

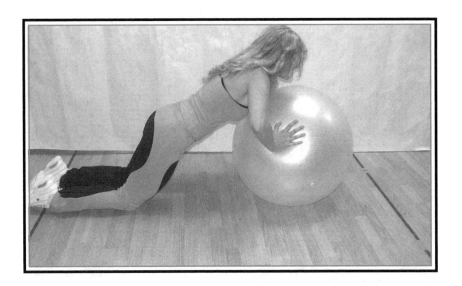

Push-Ups

Begin on hands and knees. Place the ball underneath the hips. Walk the hands out until the ball is between the knees and the ankles. Positioning the ball close to the feet increases the challenge. Place your hands on the floor, slightly wider than shoulder-distance apart. Inhale and bend your elbows, lowering the chest toward the floor. Exhale and straighten your arms, returning to start (see photos on page 18).

For a variation, place the hands on the ball and the feet on the floor as illustrated above.

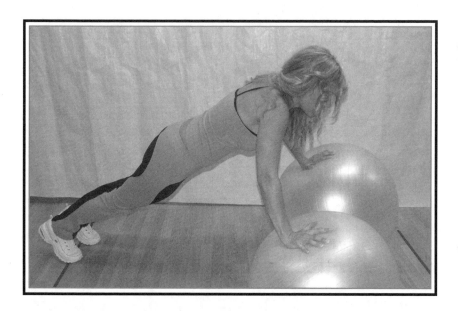

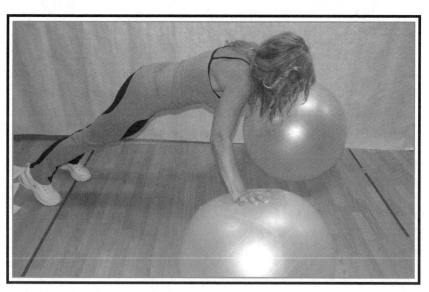

Two-Ball Pec Deck

Two balls are needed for this exercise. Kneel in front of the balls and place one hand on each. Straighten your legs behind you, pressing the toes into the floor. Inhale and slowly separate your hands, rolling the balls out to the sides. Exhale and return the balls toward each other. Keep the movement slow and controlled and use the strength of the arms and chest to stabilize the balls (see photos on page 20).

Lisa M. Wolfe

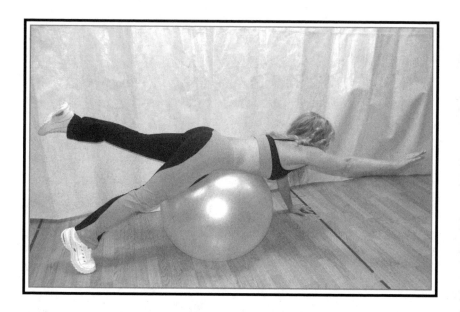

Spinal Balance

Lie face down with the ball in the center of your abdomen. Hands and feet are shoulder-width apart on the ground. To maintain this position, you may need to adjust ball size accordingly. Keep the spine in a neutral position by holding the abdominal muscles tight. Slowly raise one arm, while raising the opposite leg to hip level. Return to the starting position and repeat, using the other arm and leg. Concentrate on reaching away from your body through your fingers and toes.

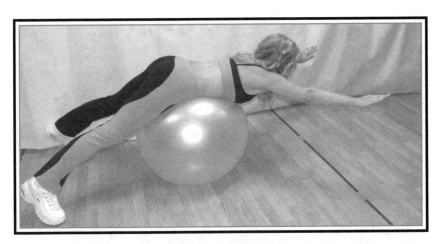

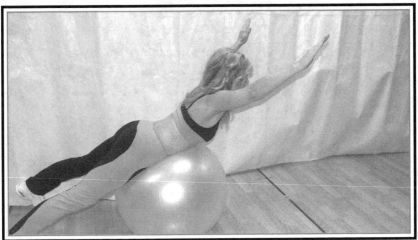

Hyperextension

Lie face down with the ball in the center of your abdomen. Straighten the legs behind the body and press the toes into the floor. Begin with arms straight out in front of you. From this starting position exhale and lift your chest off the ball while keeping your arms in the same position. Inhale and return to the starting position.

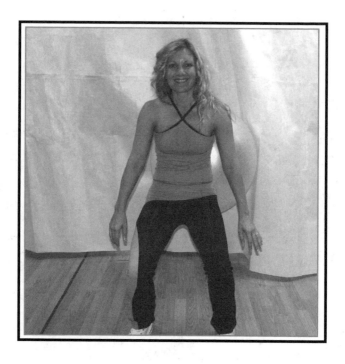

Wall Squats

Stand facing away from a wall with the ball placed between your lower back and the wall. Space your feet hip-distance apart. Inhale and bend the knees, lowering your hips toward the floor. Keep the knees over the heels and refrain from bending the knees beyond a 90-degree angle. Exhale and straighten the legs, pressing through the heels, returning to the starting position.

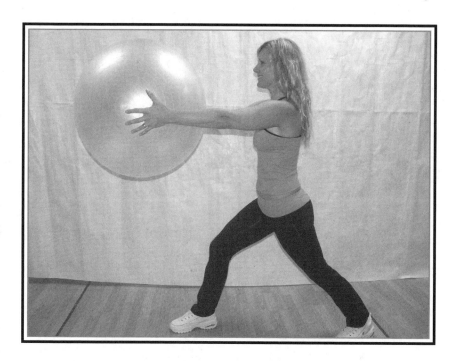

Lunge

Begin in a lunge position with the right foot approximately two feet in front of the left. Hold the ball out in front of the body. Inhale and bend the right knee to a 90-degree angle while lifting the ball overhead. Exhale and straighten the right leg while at the same returning the ball out in front of the chest. Repeat the sequence on the left leg.

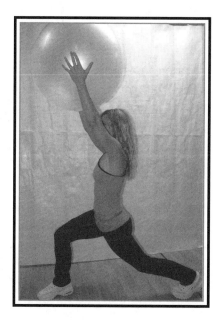

Lisa M. Wolfe

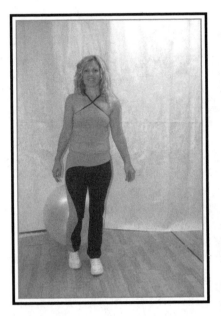 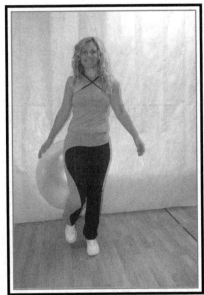

Wall Curls

Stand facing away from a wall. Place the ball on the floor next to the wall. Place your right foot on the bottom of the ball. Exhale, bend the right knee and roll the ball up the wall. Inhale and straighten the leg, stopping the ball before it touches the floor. Repeat the sequence on the left leg.

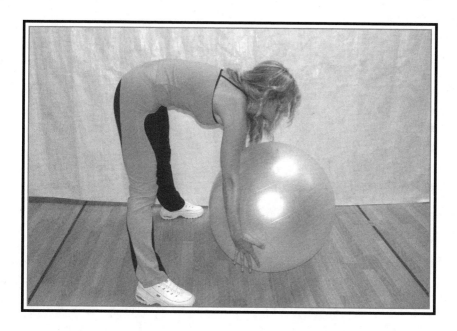

Wide Walk

Stand with your legs as wide as is comfortable. Place the ball on the floor in front of you. Bend from the waist and place your hands on the sides of the ball close to the floor. Begin walking with wide legs and rolling the ball with your fingertips. Maintain a tightened stomach as you are walking. Walk around the room for 30 to 45 seconds, rest and repeat.

Lisa M. Wolfe

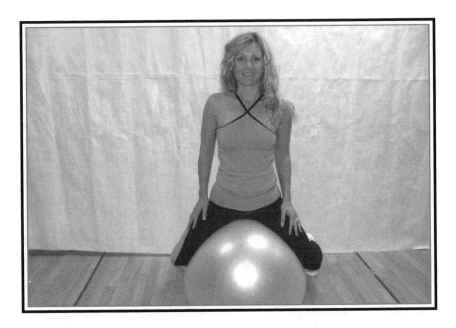

Ball Squeeze

Place the ball on the floor. Approach the ball as if you were going to straddle a horse. Sit on the ball with knees pointing toward the floor and your feet behind your body. Press your toes into the floor. You may rest your hands on the ball in between your knees for support. Exhale and squeeze the ball between your knees. Inhale and release the squeeze.

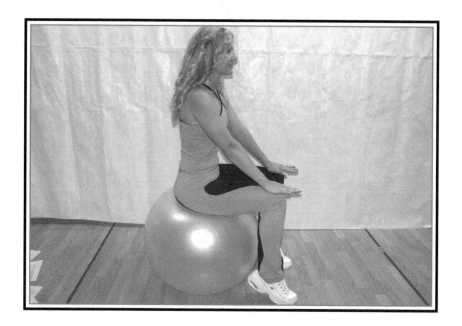

Seated Calf Raise

Sit on top of the ball with your feet on the floor. Place your hands on top of your legs just above the knees. Press down with your hands as you exhale and lift your heels off the floor. Inhale and slowly lower the heels to the floor.

Lisa M. Wolfe

Medicine Ball Exercises

A medicine ball provides a comfortable alternative to a dumbbell for strength training exercises. The outer softness of the ball adapts to any size hands and does not place stress on the joints of the fingers. The sand-filled ball is not only comfortable; it also provides intense strength training. We can maneuver the ball into alternative strengthening positions in order to build muscular improvements through a greater range of motion.

A reasonable beginning weight is 6 pounds. As strength improvements are seen, the weight of the medicine ball should be increased.

Guidelines

- Repeat 10 to 12 repetitions of each exercise.
- Perform two to three sets for maximum strength gains.
- Keep the spine straight and the stomach muscles pulled in tight.
- Maintain a firm grasp on the ball. Refrain from gripping too tightly.
- Keep a slight bend in the knees for standing exercises.
- Keep a slight bend in the elbows throughout the exercises.
- Perform exercises in a room with clear space to allow for movement.
- Listen to your body and pull back if feeling pain.

Lisa M. Wolfe

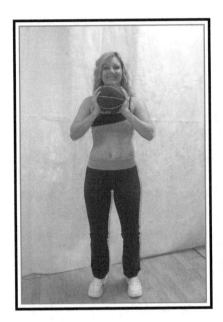 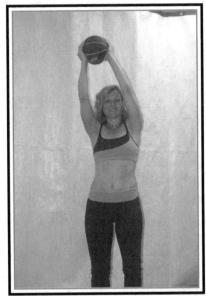

Y-Press

Stand tall with feet hip-distance apart and knees slightly bent. Grasp the medicine ball between both hands and place it in front of your chest. You will now maneuver the ball in a pattern that makes a capital letter Y. Exhale and lift the ball overhead, bringing it slightly to the right. Inhale and release the ball to the chest. Exhale and lift the ball overhead, bringing it slightly to the left. Inhale and release the ball to the chest.

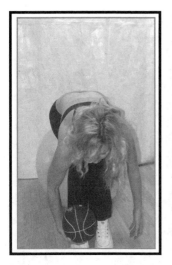 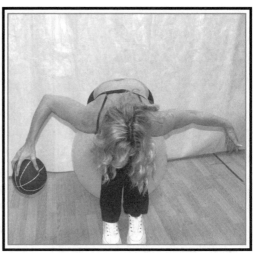

Rear Shoulder Lift

Sit with knees bent and chest folded forward onto the knees. Bend the right elbow slightly and grasp the medicine ball in the right hand. Exhale and lift the right arm out to the side, keeping the bend in the elbow. Inhale and release the arm to the starting position. Immediately transfer the ball to the left hand. Exhale and lift the left arm out to the side. Inhale and release back to the starting position. For beginners, place the opposite hand underneath the ball to assist in the lifting movement.

Lisa M. Wolfe

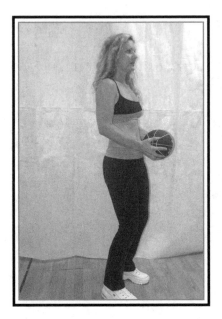 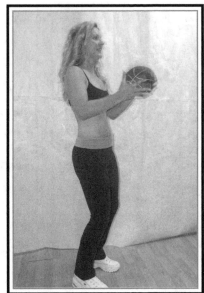

Throw and Catch

Stand tall and hold the medicine ball in your hands. Place the palms facing up and the hands underneath the ball. Hold your elbows stable into your rib cage, as if you had a belt strapping down your arms. Exhale and throw the ball in the air, keeping the arms in the tucked position. Catch the ball without moving the elbows. Inhale and lower the hands toward the hips.

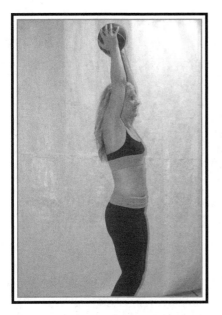 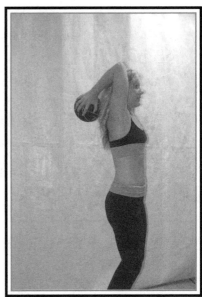

Overhead Extension

Stand tall and hold the medicine ball in both hands. Raise your arms straight over your head. Inhale and bend your elbows, lowering the hands behind the head. Keep your elbows as close to your head as possible. Exhale and straighten the arms, returning to the starting position.

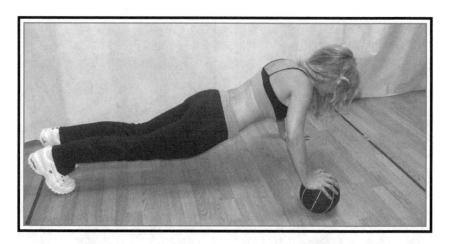

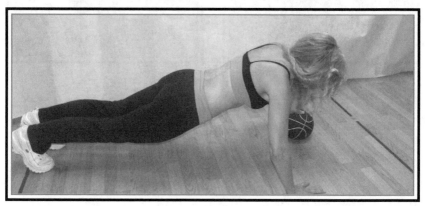

Push-Up with Roll

Kneel on your hands and knees. Place your hands on the floor approximately shoulder-distance apart. Place the medicine ball underneath one hand. Straighten your legs behind you and press your toes into the floor. Inhale, bend your elbows and lower your chest toward the floor. Exhale and straighten your arms. At the top position, roll the ball from one hand to the next. Repeat the sequence on the opposite hand.

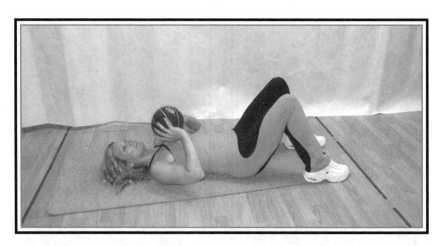

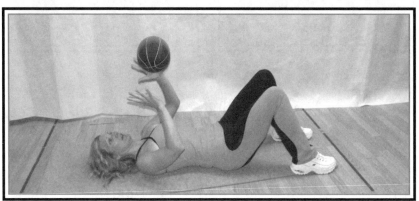

On Back — Throw and Catch

Lie on your back with your knees bent. Grasp the medicine ball in your hands. Place your hands in front of your chest and point the elbows out to the sides. Exhale, straighten your arms and throw the ball into the air. Catch the ball, inhale and bend the arms, releasing to the starting position.

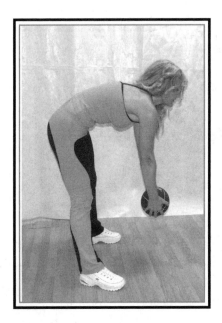 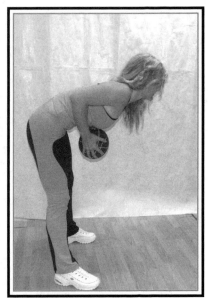

Bent Over Row

Stand with your feet hip-distance apart. Hold the medicine ball in both hands at the level of your hips. Bend forward from the waist at a 45-degree angle. Lift the arms slightly in front of the body. Exhale and pull the ball into the waist by bringing the elbows behind the body and the shoulder blades toward each other. Inhale and release the arms to the starting position.

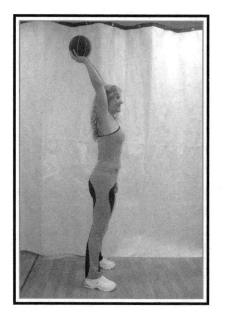 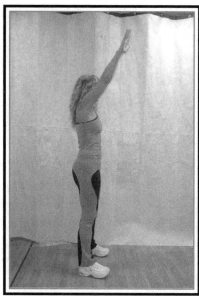

Overhead Throw

Stand tall with your feet hip-distance apart. Hold the medicine ball over your head in your right hand. Exhale and move the ball slightly toward the back of the room before moving your right arm in a throwing motion toward the floor. Release the ball straight to the floor. Repeat for repetitions and repeat on the left arm.

Lisa M. Wolfe

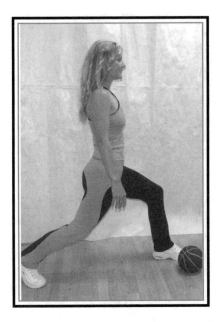 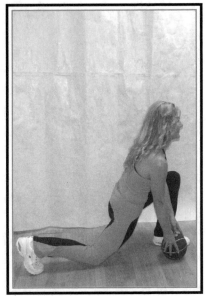

Pick-Up Lunge

Place the ball on the ground. Stand in a lunge position with the left leg forward and the right leg approximately two feet behind. Place your left foot next to the medicine ball. On an inhale bend your legs, lowering toward the floor. Reach down to pick up the medicine ball. Exhale and straighten the legs, returning to start. On the next lunge, set the ball down. Repeat for repetitions on each leg.

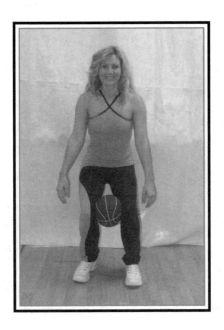

Wall Squat with Ball Between Knees

Place your back against a wall. Walk your feet away from the wall so that you are slightly leaning backward. Bend your knees no farther than 90 degrees. Place the medicine ball between your upper legs and above the knee. Keep your lower back pressed into the wall and the weight of your body rested in the heels. Hold this position for a count of 30, stand, release and repeat. Repeat sequence for three to five repetitions.

Lisa M. Wolfe

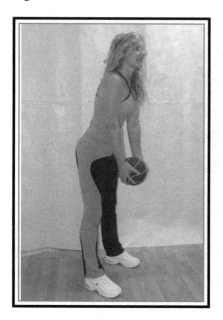 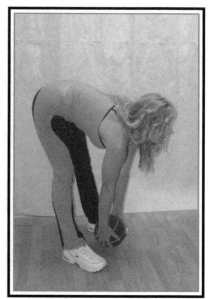

Dead Lifts

Stand tall with your feet approximately hip-distance apart. Hold the medicine ball between the hands at the level of your hips. Inhale, continue to look forward and bend from the waist, bringing the ball toward your feet. Only bend forward to a point where you can still look ahead. If the head begins to drop, pull out of the exercise. On an exhale, tighten the muscles in your backside to bring the body to the starting position.

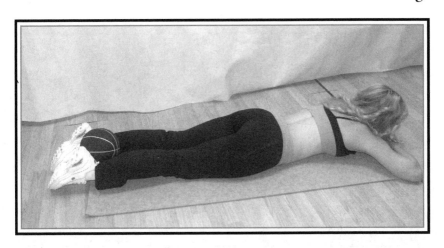

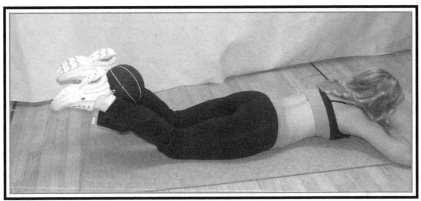

Leg Curls

Lie face down with the ball between your ankles. Bend the elbows out to the sides. Place the palms on the floor and rest the head on the backs of the hands. Exhale and bend the knees, lifting the ball off the floor. Inhale and release the ball to the starting position. When strength and coordination improve, the lift will be higher. Beginners should only lift the ball to a comfortable height.

43   Lisa M. Wolfe

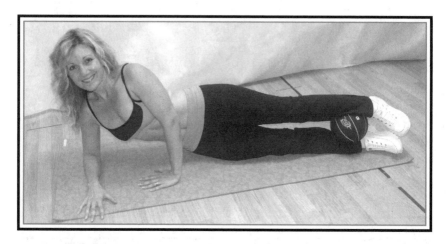

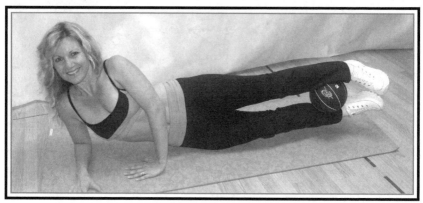

Side Lying Lift

Lie on your right side with the medicine ball between your ankles. Place your right elbow on the floor underneath the right shoulder. Stack the hips so they are one over the top of the other. Refrain from leaning backward or forward. Using the strength of your legs, exhale and lift the feet toward the sky. Inhale and release the feet to the starting position. Repeat for repetitions and repeat on the opposite leg. Beginners should place the ball between the knees.

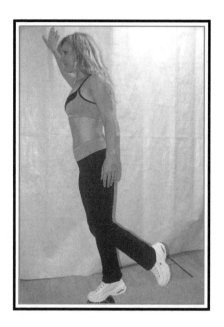

Standing Calf Raises

Place one foot on top of the medicine ball. Hang the heel off the back of the ball. Exhale and lift the heel as high as possible. Inhale and release the foot to the starting position. Repeat for repetitions and repeat on the opposite leg. Beginners should use both feet on the ball. It is also helpful to hold onto a wall or a chair.

Mini Xerball Exercises

The Mini Xerballs are an easy addition to a workout program. The soft outer shell is comfortable for the hands. The sand-filled balls provide a unique strength training alternative to dumbbells or a medicine ball. Xerballs maintain their shape, are durable and easy to clean.

Guidelines

- Repeat 10 to 12 repetitions of each exercise.
- Perform two to three sets for maximum strength gains.
- Keep the spine straight and the stomach muscles pulled in tight.
- Maintain a firm grasp on the balls, but refrain from gripping too tightly.
- Keep a slight bend in the knees for standing exercises.
- Keep a slight bend in the elbows throughout the exercises.
- Perform exercises in a room with clear space to allow for movement.
- Listen to your body and pull back if feeling pain.

Lisa M. Wolfe

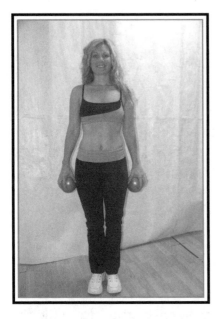

Side Lift

Stand tall with feet hip-distance apart. Grasp a ball in each hand. Place the hands next to the hips with the arms straight and the palms facing toward the body. Exhale and lift the straight arms out to the sides until parallel with the floor. Inhale and release the arms to the starting position.

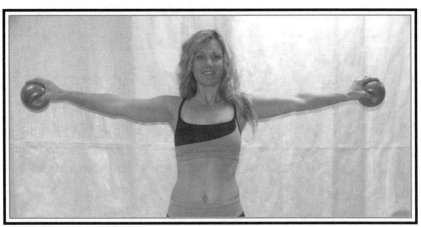

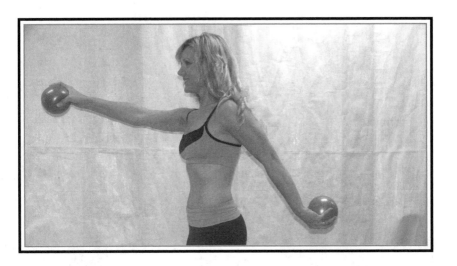

Jogging Arms

Stand tall with feet hip-distance apart and knees slightly bent. Grasp a ball in each hand. Place the hands next to the hips with the arms straight and the palms facing toward the body. Exhale and lift the right arm in front of the body and the left arm behind the body. Inhale and lower the arms to the starting position. Exhale and lift the left arm in front of the body and the right arm behind the body. Inhale and lower the arms to the starting position. Continue alternating.

Lisa M. Wolfe

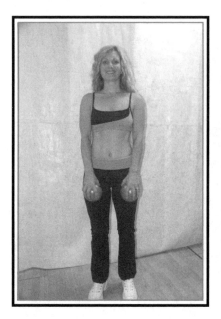 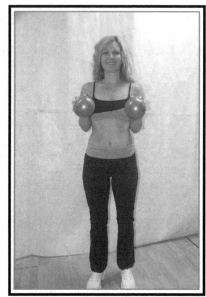

Reverse Curl

Stand tall with feet hip-distance apart. Grasp a ball in each hand. Place the hands in front of the hips with the elbows tight to the rib cage. Face the palms toward the floor. Exhale and bend the elbows, bringing the hands toward the shoulders. Inhale and release the hands to the starting position.

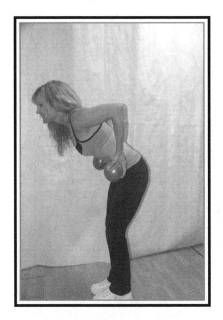 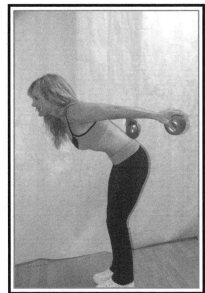

Tricep Kickback

Stand tall with feet hip-distance apart. Grasp a ball in each hand. Bend forward slightly from your waist, lifting the elbows higher than the back. Face your palms toward the front of the room. Exhale, straighten your arms and lift the balls out behind the body. The palms should now be facing toward the floor. Inhale, bend the elbows and release the hands to the starting position.

Lisa M. Wolfe

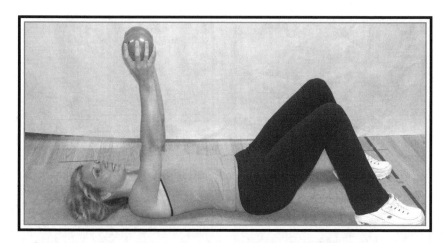

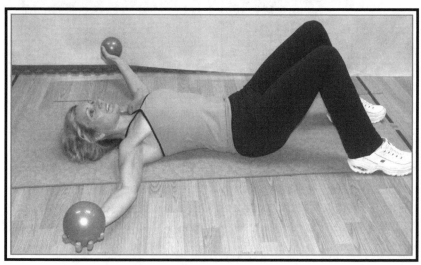

Chest Fly

Lie on your back and grasp a ball in each hand. Bend your knees and firmly press your lower back into the floor. Begin with the arms out to the sides in line with the shoulders. Exhale and bring the arms toward each other in front of the body. Keep the balls over your chest. Inhale and release the arms to the starting position (see photos on page 52).

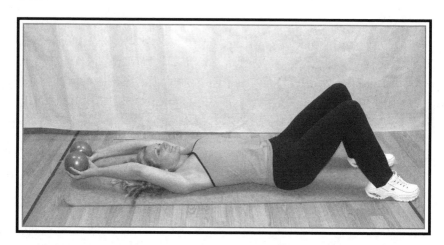

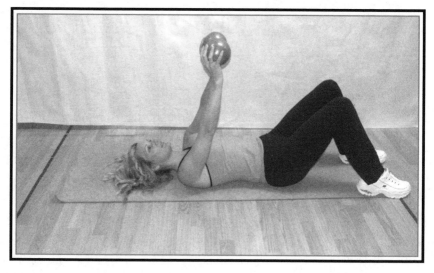

Pull-Over

Lie on your back, grasp a ball in each hand. Place straight arms over the head with the balls together. Exhale and move the arms forward until the balls are over the stomach. Inhale and extend the arms back to the starting position.

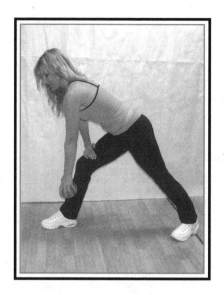 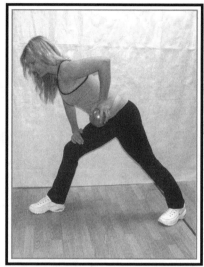

Lat Pull-In

Stand in a lunge position with the right leg approximately two feet in front of the left. Bend the right knee and place your right hand on the right thigh. Hold one or two balls in the left hand. Place the hand next to the right ankle. Exhale and lift the balls toward the left hip. Lift the elbow higher than the back. Inhale and release the balls to the starting position. Repeat with the opposite arm.

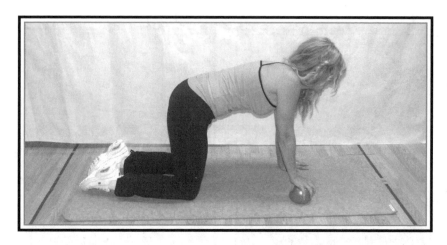

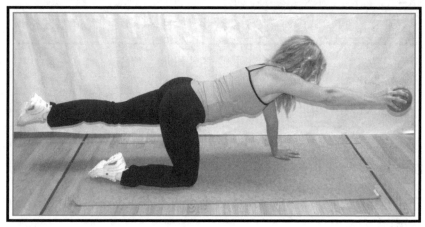

Spinal Balance

Place hands and knees on the floor. Grasp a ball in the right hand. Exhale and extend the right arm out in front of the body and the left leg behind the body. Inhale and release the arm and leg to the starting position. Repeat sequence with the opposite arm and leg.

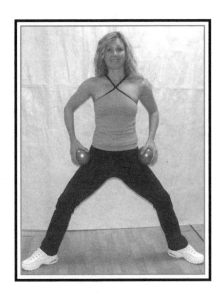 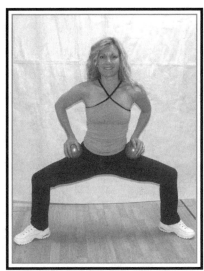

Wide Leg Squat

Stand with the legs wider than shoulder-distance apart. Bend your knees and turn your knees and toes slightly out to the sides. Grasp a ball in each hand and rest them on the tops of the legs near the hips. Inhale and bend your knees lowering your hips. Press the weight of your body through your heels. Exhale and straighten your legs, returning to the starting position.

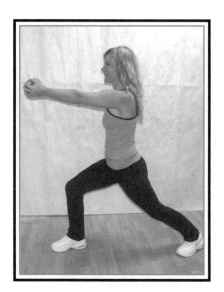 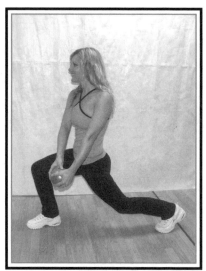

Lunge and Twist

Stand in a lunge position with the right foot approximately two feet in front of the left. Hold a ball between both hands. Extend arms straight out over the right leg. Exhale and bend the right knee, lowering the body. At the same time, gently rotate the spine, bringing the hands to the left side of the body. Keep the arms straight as you rotate. Inhale and straighten the right knee while returning the hands to the starting position. Repeat the sequence on the opposite leg.

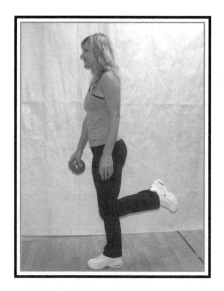 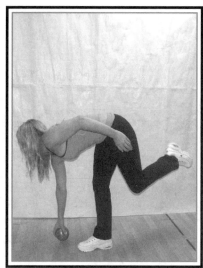

Single Leg Reach

Stand tall with the weight of the body on the right leg. Bend the left knee to lift the left foot slightly behind the body. Hold onto a ball in the right hand. Inhale and bend forward from the waist. Touch the ball to the ground. Exhale and immediately return to standing tall. Repeat the sequence on the opposite leg.

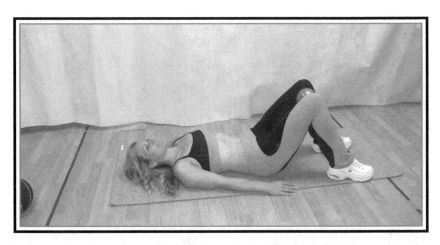

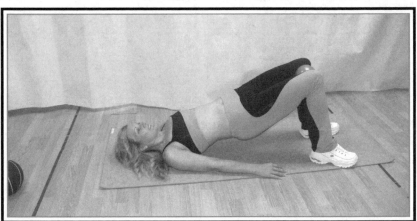

Bridge with Ball Between Knees

Lie on your back with your knees bent. Place a ball between the knees. Position the arms along the sides of your body. Exhale and lift the hips toward the ceiling, maintaining the position of the ball. Inhale and release the hips to the starting position.

The Core

The core contains muscles of the stomach and the lower back. These muscles work together to help you perform a variety of everyday movements. A strong core allows your body to function at top performance level, protects your back, aids in balance and stability, improves your posture and holds in the abdomen.

The greatest benefit to you for improving your core is that the results are seen quickly. You will feel the strength improvements after only a few workouts. You will immediately begin to enhance stability around your spine, which will improve your posture and assist in lifting activities.

As soon as the muscles of the stomach are awakened,

Core Benefits

- Improved back strength
- Increased balance and stability
- Reduced risk for back injury
- Taller posture
- Slimmer stomach

you will feel them in your everyday movements, such as turning the steering wheel of the car, closing the refrigerator door, turning to reach for a book, etc. Another benefit of core strengthening is the desire to hold the stomach in tighter. This will instantly make your stomach appear to have lost inches.

This chapter will mainly focus on the abdominal exercises, as we have covered back strengthening in the previous chapters. Refer to Chapters 3, 4 and 5 for additional back strengthening exercises.

Lisa M. Wolfe

Guidelines

- Repeat 10 to 12 repetitions of each exercise.
- Repeat two to three sets of each exercise.
- Keep the neck in line with the spine.
- Tighten the muscles of the abdomen.
- Keep the spine straight.
- Maintain proper breathing.

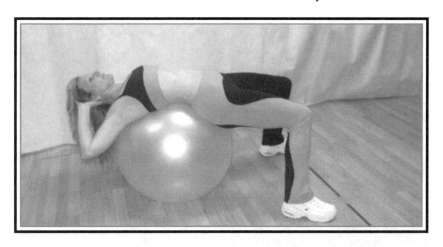

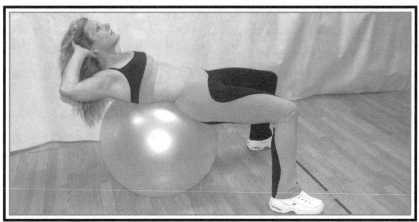

Sit-Ups

Sit on the ball and walk your feet forward until the ball is beneath the small of your back. Place your hands behind your head or crossed on top of your chest (easier option). Press your lower back into the ball. Exhale and curl the rib cage toward the pelvis. Inhale and release to the starting position. Repeat for repetitions.

Lisa M. Wolfe

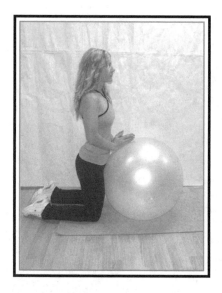

Abs Rolls

Kneel in front of the ball. Touch the ball with your legs, and place your arms in a prayer position. Place the fingertips on the part of the ball closest to you. Inhale and roll the ball away from the body using the arms to guide. In the extended position, slightly lower your hips toward the floor. At this point, only the hands should be touching the ball. Exhale and roll the ball toward the body to return to the starting position.

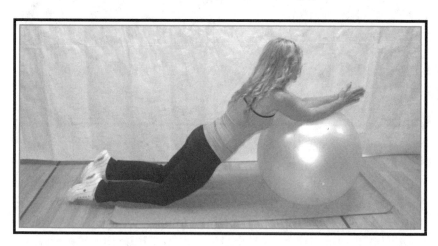

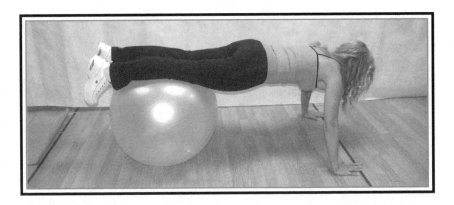

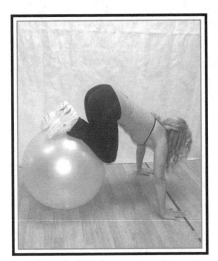

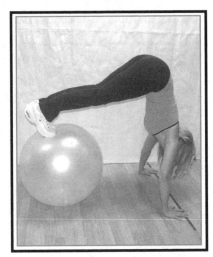

Jack Knives

Kneel on hands and knees over the top of the ball. Walk the hands away from the body, rolling the ball toward the feet. Straighten the legs with the ball positioned between the knees and the ankles. Exhale and bend the knees, rolling the ball toward the chest. Inhale and release the ball to the starting position. For an increased challenge, straighten the legs and raise the hips toward the ceiling when rolling the ball toward the chest.

Lisa M. Wolfe

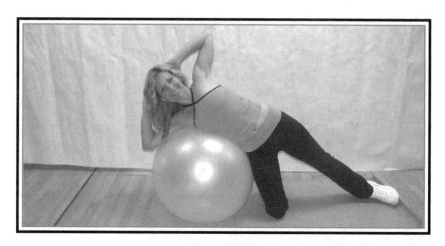

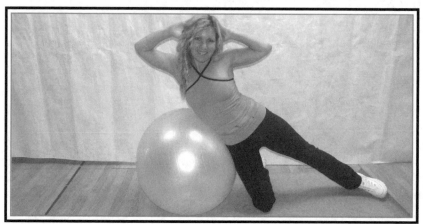

Side Lifts

Kneel on the ball next to the right hip. Shift the right hip into the ball and straighten the left leg to press the foot into the floor. Place the hands behind the head. Inhale and lengthen your right side over the top of the ball. Exhale and, using the left side, pull the body up to the starting position. Repeat for repetitions and repeat on the opposite side.

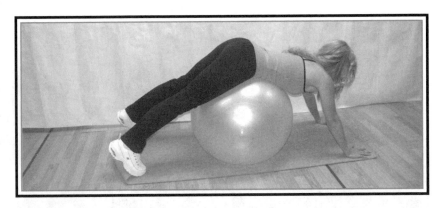

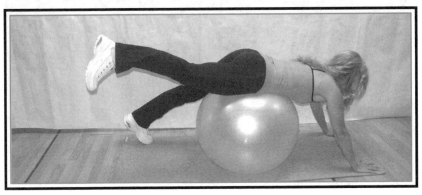

Leg Lifts

Lie face down with the ball in the center of your abdomen. Place your hands on the floor and straighten your legs slightly so your toes touch the ground. Exhale and lift one leg to hip level. Inhale and lower the leg to the floor. Repeat the lift with the opposite leg. For a more challenging exercise, lift both legs at the same time.

Lisa M. Wolfe

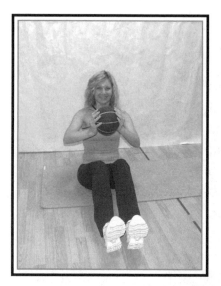 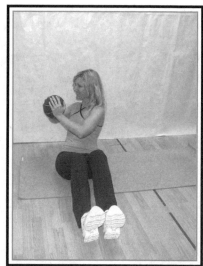

Seated Twist

Sit with your knees bent and toes pointed up toward the ceiling. Hold the medicine ball in both hands in front of your chest. Tighten your stomach and point your right elbow to the back of the room. Inhale and lower your back toward the floor. Exhale and return your body to the starting position. Inhale, point your left elbow to the back of the room and lower your back toward the floor. Exhale and return to the starting position.

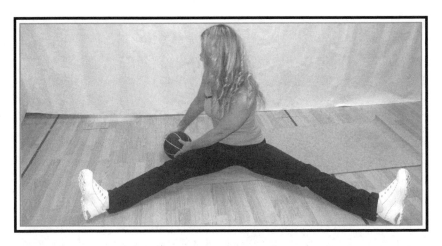

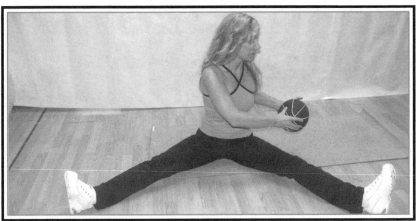

Trunk Rotation

Sit on the floor with legs spread. Place a medicine ball behind your back. Inhale and rotate to the right. Exhale and pick up the ball. Lift the ball around to your left side and replace it behind your back. Repeat for repetitions and then reverse the direction.

Lisa M. Wolfe

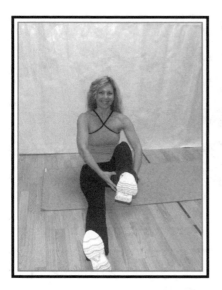 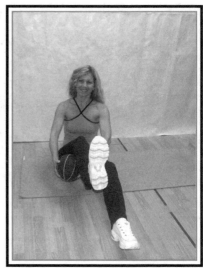

Over-Under

Sit on the floor with your legs bent. Hold a medicine ball straight in front of you. Exhale and lift your left leg and pass the ball under it from the inside. Inhale and pass it over the top of your left leg. Exhale and pass the ball under your right leg from the inside. Inhale and pass it over the top of your right leg (so the ball makes a figure eight around your legs).

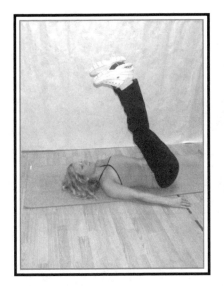 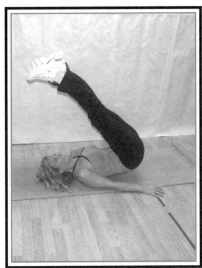

Lower Ab Lift

Lie on your back with legs extended toward the ceiling. Place a medicine ball between your ankles. Place the arms underneath your head. Exhale and lift the ball toward the ceiling by raising your hips off the floor. Inhale and release the hips to the starting position. For beginners, bend the knees and place the ball between them.

Lisa M. Wolfe

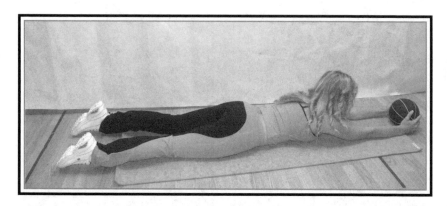

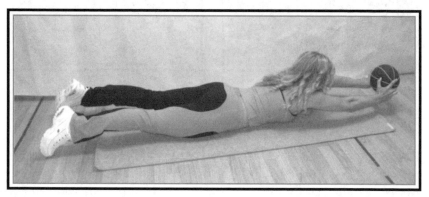

Superman

Lie on your stomach. Straighten your arms and your legs, and place a medicine ball between your hands. Exhale and lift your arms and legs off the floor. Inhale and release the body to the starting position.

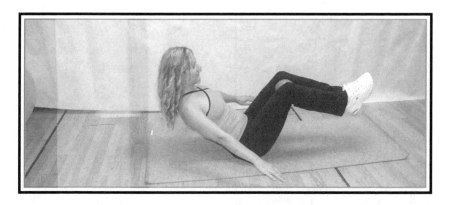

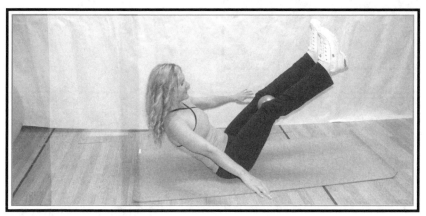

Boat

Sit on the floor with legs straight in front of you. Place a ball between the knees. Place the hands out to the sides of the body. Exhale and lift the feet off the floor. Keep the chest open and the back straight. For an advanced exercise, straighten the legs toward the ceiling. Hold for a count of 10 to 15.

Lisa M. Wolfe

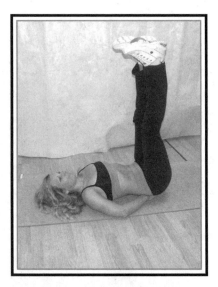

Leg Lift

Lie on your back with legs extended toward the ceiling. Place a ball between the ankles and the hands underneath the lower back. Inhale and lower the legs toward the floor to a comfortable height. Exhale and return the legs to the starting position.

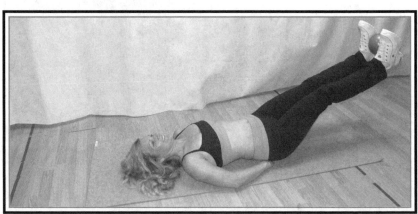

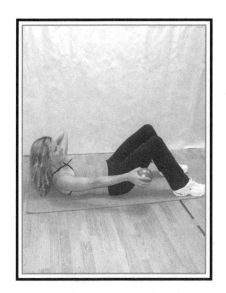 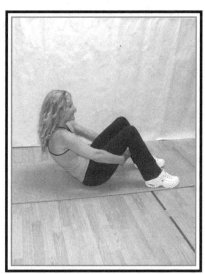

Crunch with Pass

Lie on your back with knees bent. Place the hands near the hips and hold a ball in your right hand. Exhale and lift your shoulder blades off the floor by curling the rib cage toward the hips. At the top of the movement, reach the right hand under the right leg, while at the same time reaching the left hand under the left leg. Pass the ball to the left hand. Inhale and release the body to the starting position. Repeat the movement, passing the ball from left to right.

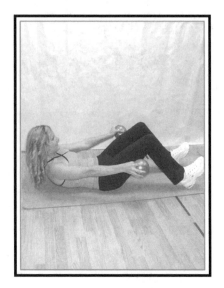 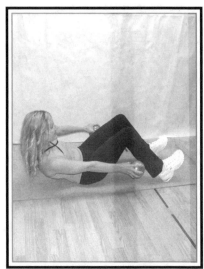

Side Reach

Lie on your back with your knees bent. Grasp a ball in each hand. Place the hands near the outside of the hips. Raise your shoulder blades off the floor. Exhale and reach the right hand toward the right ankle. Inhale and return the body to the center. Exhale and reach the left hand toward the left ankle. Inhale and return the body to the center.

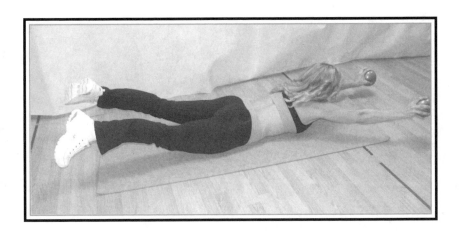

Swim

    Lie face down with arms and legs out straight. Grasp a ball in each hand. Exhale and lift the arms and legs toward the ceiling. Maintain normal breathing as you move the arms and legs up and down as if swimming. Hold for a count of 10 to 15.

Lisa M. Wolfe

Flexibility/Massage

The versatility of the stability balls provides us a wonderful tool for improving flexibility. The ball offers support when needed for those positions that are intense. The ball also increases the range of motion in a stretch for deeper flexibility gains. For those who have difficulty getting onto and up from the floor, the ball allows for an easier transition and also a variety of stretches that do not require placing the body on the floor.

Guidelines

- Hold each stretch for 15 to 30 seconds.
- Maintain normal breathing throughout the stretch.
- Keep the spine straight.
- Keep the stomach tight.
- You should feel tightness, but not pain.

Ball Benefits

- Improves flexibility
- Increases range of motion
- Allows for easier transition into stretching exercises
- Provides variety of movements
- Offers a gentle support

Lisa M. Wolfe

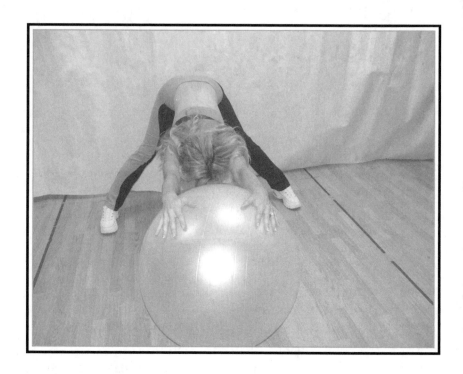

Wide Leg Stretch

Stand with legs wider than shoulder-distance apart. Place your hands on a ball in front of you. Face your heels toward the back of the room and straighten your legs to press your hips behind the body. Bend forward from the waist and rest your elbows on the ball. As you feel the stretch begin to deepen, lower the upper body toward the floor. Roll the ball away from the body and place hands on top of the ball.

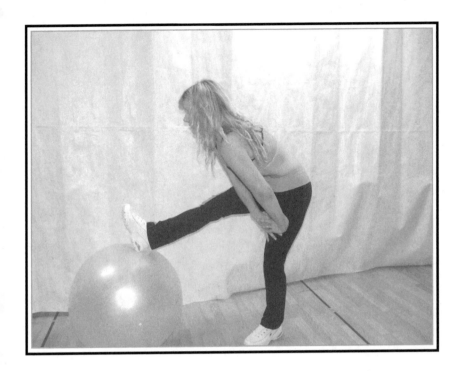

Hamstring Stretch

Stand and place the right foot on the ball. Straighten the right leg. Slightly bend the left leg and rest the hands on the left upper thigh. Slowly bend forward from the hips until a stretch is felt in the back of the right leg. Hold and repeat on the left leg.

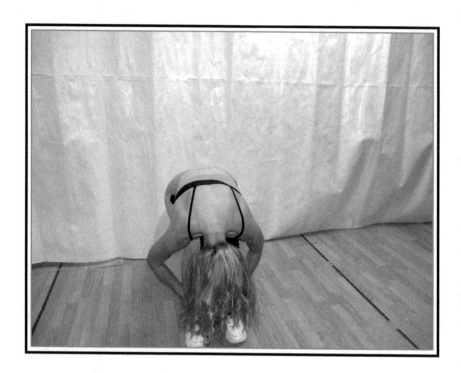

Lower Back Stretch

Sit on top of the ball. Bend your knees and place your feet directly underneath them. Fold forward from the waist bringing your chest toward your knees. Bring your hands toward the floor. Relax the neck and look down between the feet.

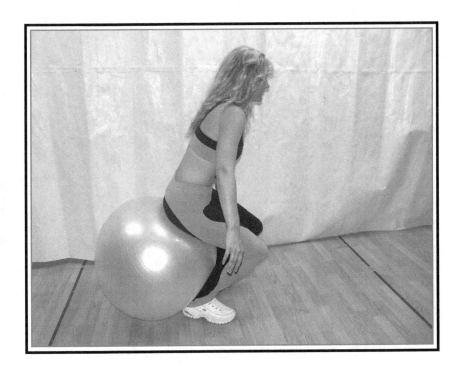

Calf Stretch

Sit on top of the ball. Bend your knees and place your feet approximately 12 inches in front of your body. Roll forward, grasping the ball with the backs of the legs. Slightly lift the ball off the floor. Press the heels toward the floor to feel the stretch.

Lisa M. Wolfe

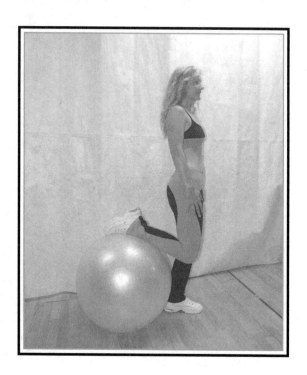

Quadriceps Stretch

Stand with the ball behind you. Bend the right knee and place the top of the right foot on the ball. Extend the right leg behind the body until a stretch is felt in the front of the right leg. Hold and repeat on the left leg.

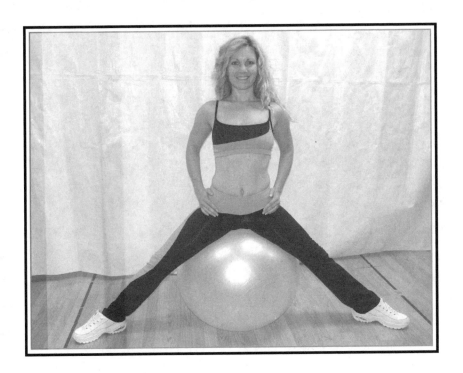

Seated Inner Thigh Stretch

Sit on top of the ball. Widen your legs out to the sides. Keep your knees straight and position your knees and toes toward the sides of the room.

Lisa M. Wolfe

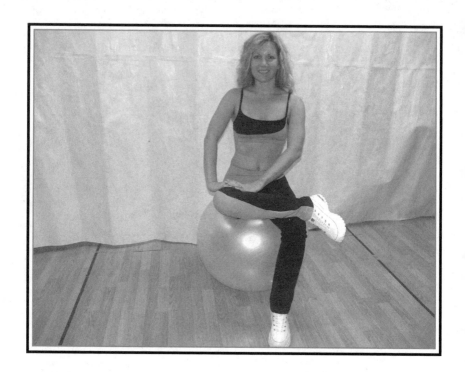

Seated Hip Stretch

Sit on top of the ball. Place the right foot on the left knee. Place the hands on the right inner thigh. Gently press the thigh toward the floor. Hold and repeat on the left leg.

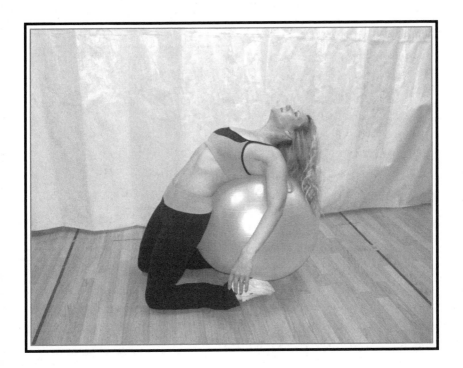

Camel Stretch

Kneel on the floor and place the ball on the backs of the legs. Using the hands to guide, slowly bend backwards, resting the back on the ball. Keep the neck in line with the spine and look slightly upward. Hold for a count of 10.

Tennis Ball Massage

A tennis ball is an incredible tool to use for your own personal massage. The ball can provide relief for tight muscles after a workout, or anytime. The best time to perform this technique is after the body is warm and you have spent time with your flexibility exercises.

The massage has a simple basis for its effectiveness. You place the ball on the part of the body that is tight, rest your weight on it and hold for pressure release. Attempt to hold the ball in position for one minute. If the pain worsens, release immediately and seek medical attention.

Ball Benefits

- Provides daily massage
- Portable
- Eases stress
- Reduces fatigue
- Reduces muscular tension

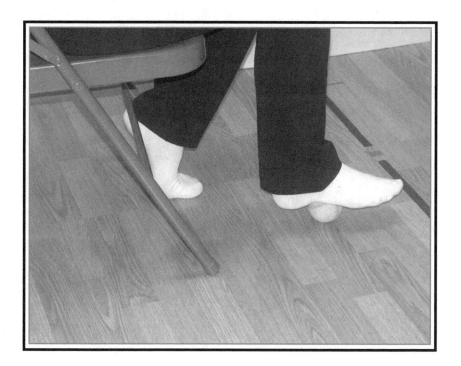

Feet

Sit in a chair and place the ball under your foot. Gently roll the foot back and forth until relief is felt. Repeat on both feet.

Lisa M. Wolfe

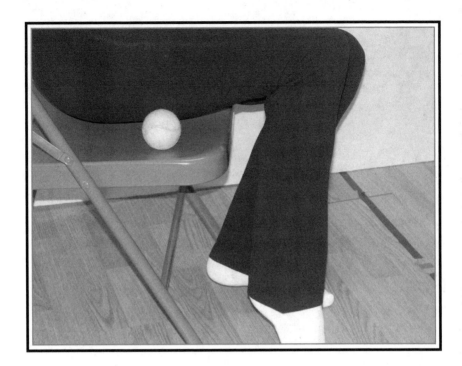

Hamstrings

Sit in a chair. Place the ball near your sit bone. Roll the ball to the place on the back of the leg where you feel the most discomfort. Rest your weight on the ball, shifting to increase or decrease the amount of pressure. Repeat on both legs.

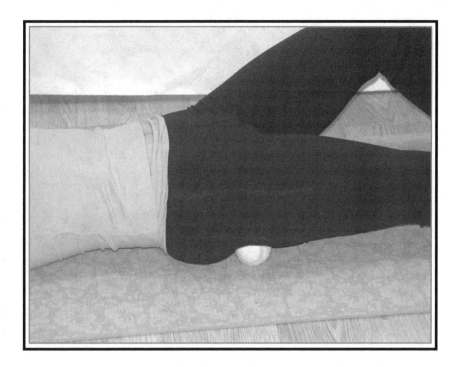

Gluteus

Lie on your back with legs straight and arms at the sides. Place a ball in the center of the buttock. Position the ball to where you feel the most discomfort. Rest your weight on the ball, shifting to increase or decrease the amount of pressure. Repeat on both sides.

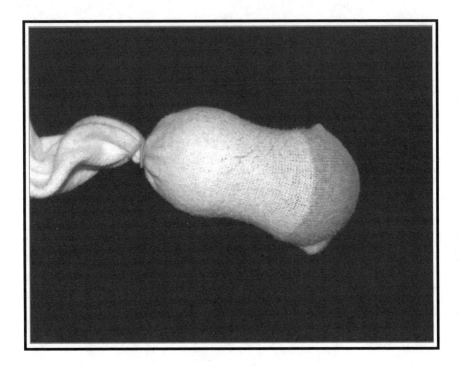

Back

Place two tennis balls into a sock. Secure the end with a rubber band. Lie on your back with knees bent. Place the balls on either side of the base of your spine. The balls should not be directly on the spinal column. Breathe normally as you inch the balls up your spine. If you feel any particular tight areas, rest the balls in that position until you feel a release. Continue to roll the balls up the spine until you reach the shoulder blades.

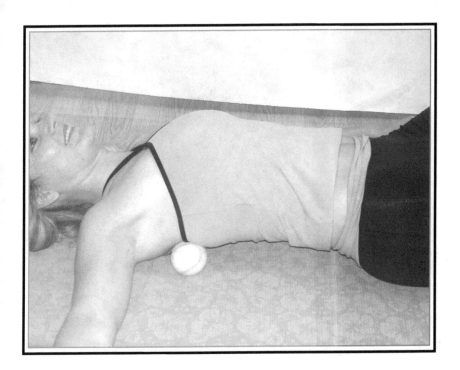

Shoulders

Lie on your back with knees bent. Place a tennis ball underneath the top of the left shoulder, near the joint. Lift your hips toward the ceiling to increase the amount of pressure on the ball. Elevate or release your hips in response to the pain. Repeat on the right side.

Lisa M. Wolfe

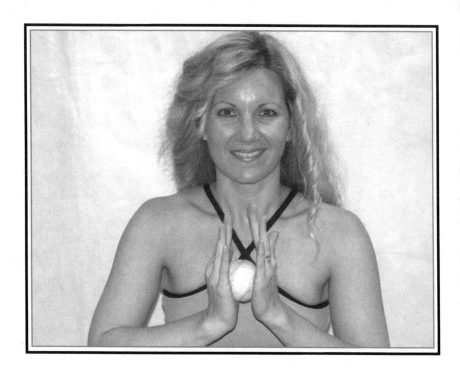

Hands

Sit and hold a tennis ball between the palms. Position the fingers toward the ceiling. Roll the ball between the hands, feeling the release of tension.

Special Considerations

While the balls are adaptable to most everyone, certain precautions still exist:

- Before beginning any exercise program, it's important to check with your doctor.
- Wear proper clothing and shoes for the activities.
- Follow the ball manufacturer's guidelines exactly to avoid overinflating the stability balls.
- Adequately hydrate and fuel your body throughout the day.
- Rest a day in between strength training workouts.
- Clear the room for ease of motion.

For those with:

- Hypertension, reduce the amount of weight and relax your grip on the balls.
- Back pain, keep the knees bent throughout the exercises and avoid overextending the spine.
- Pregnancy, please check with your doctor before beginning this or any exercise program. Do not lie on your back for abdominals or other strengthening exercises.
- Shoulder injuries or dislocations, avoid overhead lifting with the weight. Use a lighter weight amount.
- Wrist pain, carpal tunnel syndrome, or arthritis in the hands, rest on the knuckles instead of the palms in spinal balance, jack knives, and push-ups. Keep wrists as straight as possible throughout the exercises.

Lisa M. Wolfe

- Joint injuries, rest until the joint has completely healed.
- Balance issues, use the stability ball in increments until your awareness improves.
- Have latex or rubber allergies, check with the manufacturer.

For More Information

To purchase balls and equipment:
- Fitness Wholesale www.fitnesswholesale.com 800-396-7337
- SPRI www.spriproducts.com 800-222-7774
- Simple Fitness Solutions www.simplefitnesssolutions.com 888-283-0292

For an excellent —
- Stability ball video workout:www.patrickgoudeau.net
- Medicine ball video: www.jumpinc.com
- Mini Xerball video: www.yo-wei.com

To purchase clothing seen in this book:
- www.fitcouture.com

To reach Lisa with questions or comments: www.yogaband.com

Lisa M. Wolfe